I0417224

# Chronicles of Afro-dite:
## Escaping the Tangled Web Of Weava

A Novel
by Amirah Bellamy

Illustrations by Artabulous and Jabari Bellamy

# Chronicles of Afro-Dite:
## Escaping the Tangled Web Of Weava

*is dedicated to the sleeping Divine Ones on the quest to re-discovering Self.*

# Acknowledgments

*I thank my spirit guides of the fairy realm for instilling within me creativity, humility, peace, love and the beauty of fond childhood memories.*

# TABLE OF CONTENTS

# One

Long, long ago on a planet far, far away called Sirius lived a goddess named Afro-dite. Afro-dite was the beautiful daughter of a powerful creator named Rah. Rah was grandfather to the titans and great-grandfather to the gods.

He was what was called a primordial being. This meant that he was one of the most highly evolved beings in existence. Only the divine ones were evolved enough to see him. For this reason Rah was known throughout all of existence as the Hidden One. In fact, none other than his wife, daughter and a very special select few gods and goddesses could perceive him.

He was unlike anything that many humans could perceive. Many simply described him as consciousness. He represented the highest level of evolution that the human mind could perceive, yet that was not to say that he wasn't even more evolved than that.

Rah was not a being that had been birthed as birthing was a human concept. Rah and the other primordial beings merely thought themselves into existence. There were other primordial beings aside from Rah. Collectively they were all considered to be one being or force that was indivisible.

Nonetheless, Rah was considered the most powerful of all creators. Though with all of his power Rah had a soft spot and was his beloved daughter Afro-dite. He loved her immensely and as a result he literally gave her the world.

Afro-dite was absolutely beautiful in the eyes of anyone who looked upon her, including her dad. She was the color of the sands of time and her smile was bright enough to bring about the light of day.  In fact, her father always said that she was the eye of Rah.  Through her eyes one could see all of creation.

Yet, it was her hair that was her most admirable trait.  She was even named after her beautiful hair.  Afro-dite wore her hair in the most charming afro that upon seeing would stop one dead in their tracks.  It was a black, tightly coiled, larger than life, shiny, radiant spectacle of beauty that simply made her radiate.

Nonetheless, even with all of her beauty, a father who had given her the world and a world of beings who worshipped her, Afro-dite still longed for something more.  She always felt like something was missing and that she just wanted to do something that brought meaning to her life.  Afro-dite had a longing and that was to be sent on a mission by her father.

She grew bored having nothing more to

do than rule the beings of her planets. Besides that she began to feel that her world was just too boring and so she wanted to spend some time in a more exciting world, one with some real action.

She often grew frustrated watching her father send all the other gods and goddesses out on exciting missions, many of whom were a lot less powerful than she. She wanted to prove herself worthy of her father's belief in her. She wanted to do something to make him proud. So when her millionth birthday came around she thought it was the perfect opportunity to ask her dad for the one thing that would make her happy.

# Two

Waking up that morning felt like the best day in the world to Afro-dite.  It was a day that she had been looking forward to for what seemed like lifetimes.  She was beaming from ear to ear as she bounced around off of the stars with a smile bright enough to light up the universe.

"Good morning dad!  Do you know what today is?" Afro-dite greeted beaming from ear to ear.

"Hmmm…. let me think," Rah said with a sly grin as he knew already what Afro-dite was planning to ask of him for the 20 millionth time.

"Dad are you serious?  You don't know what today is?  It's a very special day.  In fact, you've always said that it's THE most special day of your life!" Afro-dite exclaimed.

"Hmmmm is that so? I can't imagine what in my creations that could be," Rah said half smiling.

"Dad! Come on! You *must* know what today is. It's only been your favorite day, your favorite celebration, your favorite reason for throwing the most grand party of all parties for the last *million* years!" Afro-dite said growing a bit agitated.

"Ooooohhh!!! THAT! Wow is it already that time! My how time flies. Seems we just celebrated your birthday sunshine" Rah said smiling at Afro-dite warmly.

"Yeah dad it's my birthday and it's the big one! I can't wait to see what you got me! So what is it? What did you get me dad? Is it a mission this time?" Afro-dite inquired with one raised eyebrow.

Rah smiled as he gazed at his beautiful daughter wanting so much to grant her wish, but still feeling that she wasn't yet ready. "I guess you'll have to wait and see at the party sunshine," Rah said being mysterious.

"Oh come on dad. Just give me a hint? I'll still act surprised at the party, I promise," Afro-dite begged.

"Nope and I promise it'll be all the better if you wait and see later at the party. In fact, I think that you should go and get ready as should I. I'll see you later sunshine," Rah said stopping to kiss his daughter on the cheek adoringly as he sped off trying to avoid any further questioning from his 'detective' daughter.

"I sure hope you're right dad, but if it's not a mission I'm afraid I won't be happy *at all*," Afro-dite shouted after him.

Afro-dite knew that her father still had his doubts about sending her off on a mission. She was his only child and he was always very protective of her. All the same she was also very powerful and there wasn't too much in existence that could stand up against her. Thus, she just didn't understand why he couldn't trust that she was ready and could take care of herself. After all she wasn't exactly a little girl anymore. She was turning one million years old!

Afro-dite was deep in thought about how wonderful it would be to finally be sent on a mission. She pictured herself going on the most exciting mission imaginable too, one that was absolutely action packed. She knew that she could do it. She just needed to be given the chance.

The more she thought about it the more confident she grew that her father would grant her wish and that she would finally get to see her dream come true. Getting more excited by the moment, Afro-dite went to go get ready for the biggest party of her lifetime.  She couldn't wait for the fun to begin.

# Three

Finally, the time had arrived for Afro-dite's birthday party! Everyone who was anyone in creation was in attendance. Afro-dite looked absolutely amazing. She wore a long, flowing gown made of stars that lit up the universal skies and made Afro-dite glisten.

The party was held on the rooftop of Rah's palace and he pulled out all the stops to make it the party of the megaannum. There were stars spelling out "Happy Birthday Afro-dite!!" There was a signature drink being served that shined like the sun, which Rah named "Afro-sun". The floors were made of diamonds and beneath them beautiful lights glowed like the aurora borealis.

There was a giant birthday cake made of

the essence of Rah. When Afro-dite blew out the candles her father's essence scattered everywhere instantly sprouting into thousands of beautiful blue morpho butterflies. To put it simply, the palace was a vision taken from the book of heaven.

Rah also had the best in entertainment. There were musicians who played music in the key of all sounds blissful, which instantly put attendees in a state of peace. Rah had also gotten the best of the best of magicians in all of creation to perform the most mind-blowing magic tricks ever before seen.

There was one magic trick in particular that both amazed and struck Afro-dite as odd. Using some type of mind control ability the magician managed to get into the minds of all of the guests including Rah, Afro-dite and her mother, Amaunet. He then created an alternate reality where the primordials, titans and gods were all turned into humans living on the planet Saturn in a past time.

Everyone's body had been transformed, all but the magician. Having seen themselves in human form they were all for a moment caught off guard. Tension began to fill the air and some of the Titans and gods began to attack the magician.

"What is this magic? Change us back this instant!" the Titan Cleophus demanded.

"Oh let the magician do his little tricks," Rah chimed in unconcerned.

"So what are we to do with these bodies magician?" an unidentifiable voice yelled from the crowd.

"Love, laugh and be merry," the magician cheered as the surroundings began to transform again.

Just then, before anyone else could comment they were transported to the planet

Mars.  Being on Mars didn't sit well with any of the guest who seemed to be a bit rattled.

"I demand that you change us back this instant magician.  There is nothing entertaining about this trick," the Titan Tyrese snapped.

Then before the magician could respond several armored warriors appeared instantly out of nowhere and came charging toward the guests.  The warriors had the most horrifying faces.  Their eyes were literally made of blood, they had web-like looking hair and appeared have super-human abilities.

The guest grew agitated as they were dissatisfied with the unfair advantage that the warriors had over them as they were still stuck in human form.  There definitely was not a level playing field as the guest were all devoid of any powers, weapons or any other means of protecting themselves.

Afro-dite looked around in puzzlement

unable to determine whether the whole thing was actually part of what her father planned for her party or not.  If is was it was very out of character for him.  Besides that, none of the party guests seemed the least bit amused.

Just then the planet began to quake and the guests began running around frantically seeking shelter on the uninhabited planet. There were no signs of life currently on the planet so the guests didn't know what to do.  It had been lifetimes since they'd been on Mars and had forgotten the layout of the planet, especially in their panicked state.

Afro-dite became less and less amused by the magician's tricks as did many of the party guests.  She looked at Rah who still seemed rather unmoved so Afro-dite was still unable to discern whether the magician's trick was planned or not.  She couldn't imagine that her father would think that such a trick would be amusing to her.  So she concluded the trick was of the magician's own doing.

Whatever, the case she grew tired of the trick and it would soon end. Meanwhile, the guests, all with the exception of the primordial ones were running around panicking and acting out as humans as things got a lot worse before they got better.

# Four

Feeling trapped by the weaknesses of their mortal bodies the guests became overwhelmed with feelings of fear as they were powerless to defend themselves. Screams began to ring from the crowd and chaos followed as many began running around madly seeking out an escape.

The air was thick with fear and tension. No one knew quite how to respond. Many were uncertain about the extent of the illusion. So they didn't know if the human bodies could actually get hurt. They also didn't know whether the warriors posed an actual threat or if what happened in the illusion would transfer back to their own reality.

So many ran in fear of the unknown.

Then if matters couldn't get any worse out of the skies came the biggest giant that any of them had ever seen.

Most strange was that out of all the guests, the titans seemed the most unsettled. Meanwhile the gods were unusually calm. Then, as expected, though things worsened the primordials didn't seem at all threatened.

The titans, who were panic-stricken demanded that the magician end the illusion immediately. So finally, after seeing that many of the guests were not at all amused by the magic trick and seeing that it had gone far enough the magician ended the illusion and everything was returned back to normal.

"What magic was that?" demanded several of the guests all shouting at Rah having a momentary lapse of judgement as to who they were speaking to.

Rah was never to be challenged in such

a way and everyone in existence knew better than to speak to him in such a disrespectful manner.

"Watch your tongue children!" Rah ordered slightly annoyed with the vibration of his voice sending a ripple through all of existence.

All were instantly calm and silent. It didn't take long for everyone to collect themselves as it was always best not to tempt one's fate with Rah.

Noticing that it was probably best to stop with any further tricks the magician turned to Rah, bowed and then did the same to Afro-dite and her mother before turning to exit the party.

Then, just as fast, as if nothing had occurred the party guests went back to enjoying the party, socializing, eating and being merry.

"Wow dad! That musician sure was *interesting*.... Was he a magician of your creation? " Afro-dite observed.

"No dear, that magician was a gift from Cleophus. I did think him odd as well. Very odd indeed," Rah said trailing off looking at Cleophus deep in thought.

Cleophus was Rah's grandchild and a titan. He and Afro-dite weren't particularly close so she thought his gift quite strange. More than that she really didn't know him to be much of the gift giver. Cleophus was always quite the quiet one. He wasn't much of a prankster.

Afro-dite also remembered how agitated he seemed about the magic trick, which didn't quite make sense. The whole thing was rather mysterious and Afro-dite definitely wanted to know more about what it all meant.

Not sure what to make of any of it Afro-dite went back to mingling with her party guest and enjoying her big day. She figured that the answers would come at a later time. Though she also planned to do some more investigating. The same seemed true for Rah as he stared on at Cleophus deep in thought.

# Five

Though Afro-dite thought the whole magic trick part of the party very odd she was delighted with the way that the rest of her party turned out.  For the remainder of the party she was on cloud Rah.  However, she was still anxious to see what huge gift her father had to present to her for her birthday.  So she anxiously awaited the moment of truth.

Then as if reading her mind, Rah called on everyone's attention for the announcement of Afro-dite's birthday gift.  Quickly, everyone gathered.  When Rah spoke, *everyone* listened.  From the largest to the tiniest of creatures all quickly came over to gather around Rah's table to hear the big announcement.

Afro-dite's mother, Amaunet stood next

to her husband Rah looking as radiant as ever. To all it was clear who Afro-dite got her beauty from. If Afro-dite was the definition of beauty then Amaunet was clearly it's mother because beauty didn't even begin to describe what she was.

Amaunet, like Rah, was also a primordial being. As a couple Rah and Amaunet were the definitions of soulmates. Together they formed the primordial ocean. They were each what completed the other. They warmed the hearts of all who had the opportunity to gaze upon the beauty of their love.

Amaunet had skin that glistened and was as smooth as an ocean bed. Her eyes were most alluring and like her daughter her hair was her most admired feature. Amaunet had the fluffiest head of shiny curls that seemed to smile and glide across space and time extending for miles and miles making it impossible for anyone without a magical means to stand next to her.

As Amaunet looked on at her daughter adoringly awaiting her husband's announcement she enjoyed a flashback of all the fond memories of Afro-dite's prior birthdays. Gazing upon Afro-dite, Amaunet wondered how her daughter had grown up so fast.

Amaunet knew already of Rah's planned gift to Afro-dite. It was a gift to rival all others and she was anxious to see the look on Afro-dite's face when Rah revealed the highly anticipated birthday gift.

Finally, it was the moment that Afro-dite had been waiting for and she was bursting at the seams with excitement as she listened on. It seemed that she'd been waiting for that moment her entire life.

She was certain that she was finally going to get her first mission. She envisioned that the mission might be something exciting and that it would be her chance to prove herself to her dad.  She wanted a chance to carry on the family reputation of being the most powerful ones.  She wanted a chance at greatness.

# Six

It seemed the words couldn't make it out of her father's mouth soon enough for Afro-dite. She had to fight with everything in her might not to disrespectfully rush him along.

Everyone had gathered around and had by then settled down. It was quiet enough to hear a planet rotating. Afro-dite was on the edge of her skin. Then, as her dad began to speak she held her breath with anticipation.

"I thank you all for joining us in the celebration of the most blessed event in existence, my beautiful daughter's millionth birthday. As I look at you tonight I see that you are growing up to be so much more than even *I* ever imagined my dear. You are the goddess that all others should strive to be," Rah said gazing into Afro-dite's eyes.

Afro-dite melted as she listened on. Her father said the most beautiful things about her. She was truly a daddy's girls and she always thought herself the luckiest girl in existence. Her father moved the universe to make her happy and for that she was eternally grateful.

"So it is my honor tonight to present to my dearest daughter a birthday gift to rival all others," Rah continued before looking over at Afro-dite with the softness that no other but she ever saw. With that Rah made the long awaited announcement.

"For your millionth birthday gift my dearest daughter I give you my sunlight!" Rah roared, his voice echoing far out into the distance.

The entire room gasped in shock. No one could believe the extent of Rah's love for his daughter for bestowing such a gift upon her. His sunlight was the core of who he was and for him to gift it to his daughter was more than anyone expected.

Instantly whispers flooded the room as everyone looked on for Afro-dite's response. Yet, to everyone's surprise Afro-dite's faced was dressed in utter disappointment.

Taking notice of his daughter's less than desired response Rah went to Afro-dite and asked, "Is there something wrong my dear? Is this gift not to your liking? Why do you look so sad my child?"

Struggling to keep her composure and trying her best to choose her words wisely so as not to disrespect her father Afro-dite responded, "Father I have the deepest gratitude for your gift. However, it is not what I expected. For so long I have waited and rather patiently I might add to receive the gift of your belief in me. That is, for me, the gift that will truly rival all others."

"Yes, my dear and the gift of my sunshine is exactly that. It is I who makes the sun to shine throughout the galaxy and with that comes the greatest of responsibilities," Rah answered.

"Yes father, but that is your desire and not mines. I want to explore other worlds. I want to go on a mission and prove to you and myself the greatness of my power. I need to do that away from you and mother. Taking on the gift of your sunshine does not allow me that opportunity and only keeps me stuck here still under your close watch unable to stand on my own. I'm ready father. I can do it," Afro-dite explained.

"My dear child I more than anyone know well of your powers. I created you. It's not my distrust of your powers or your abilities to stand on your own that is of concern to me. It is that I do not think that you are ready for what comes along with that. It takes millions of years before one is ready for such things. You are still quite young and you will have plenty of time for those things. This gift will prepare you for that," Rah reasoned hoping to have gotten through to his daughter.

Seeing that Afro-dite could not be convinced of her father's well intentioned gift Amaunet intervened. "Daughter this is a gift that even I haven't been granted the honor of receiving. It is a gift that shows that your father actually *does* have a great deal of trust in your ability. Is it your father's belief in yourself that you question or your own?" Amaunet asked.

Taking a moment to contemplate her mother's question Afro-dite became overcome with embarrassment. Looking at all the eyes staring at her she bolted out of the room. Not wanting to be followed she thought herself teleported to her favorite hideaway where she always went to get away from everyone to think.

# Seven

When Afro-dite wanted to be alone she would always go to an isolated forest located on one of her worlds, which she named Majestic. The Majestic Forest was cloaked by magic that even her father could not get through.

It wasn't a typical forest. The trees there weren't made up of leaves and branches, but were instead made up of tree shaped coils of Afro-dite's hair. Afro-dite created it as a place for her to recharge.

As Afro-dite's hair was the source of much of her power there were times when she wanted to give those powers a boost. So the trees in the Majestic Forest were created for that purpose.

Afro-dite had infused the trees with both her father and mother's essence and so the energetic force of the trees was quite powerful. She also infused the trees with her own magnetic force.

Whenever Afro-dite would go to the forest, from the moment she entered it the trees would all yield to her then instantly connect to her hair. There was a tree for each strand of her hair so it created what appeared to be an extension of her hair giving her hair the appearance of being larger than life.

No one else knew about it and secretly Afro-dite had made it as a place to try out some of her new powers, which she'd also developed in secret. One of the reasons why she so badly wanted to be assigned to a mission was that she wanted to test some of her powers out. She'd been perfecting them for millenniums.

As the daughter of two primordial parents Afro-dite was born with several powers, which included destruction, teleportation, energy reading, magnetism and shape-shifting. Then on her own she also developed two additional powers, which included the power to heal using the oils produced from her hair and command over the elements.

As she walked through the forest with her shoulders slumped over in disappointment having lost the regal posture that she held just moments earlier at her party she thought about all that she could do if only given the chance to go on a mission. She was more than ready and she was so upset that her father did not believe in her. She'd done everything that she could to convince him and she was tired of campaigning for herself.

If he didn't believe in her enough she resolved that she'd just have to find another way. So she sat for decades in the Majestic Forest trying to come up with a way to do just that.

Meanwhile, back at Sirius Rah grew more and more ill as the result of the departure of his daughter. She had never run off like that. He had everyone looking for her and no one could find any trace of her. It was as if she'd disappeared.

All the while seeing Rah in a weakened state upon the loss of his daughter others close to him began to plot ways to attack him. Because of his power Rah was both admired and envied. So there was always someone waiting to take his place. Thus, with his daughter gone many thought it the perfect opportunity to strike.

Sensing the plots against him, Rah began sending those close to him who he suspected of such plots away on missions to keep them both occupied and away from him while he figured out a way to defend himself.

He'd heard that some among the gods were teaming up with the demi-gods and humans of one of his planets called Earth to combine forces to take him down. So though upset over the whereabouts of his daughter he was even more troubled over the betrayal of those whom he'd trusted and loved.

By day he travelled the galaxy skies deep in thought about what to do. By night he pondered his own plan of attack on those who plotted against him.

Rah knew that with power came such things and that having such powers would often make him vulnerable to such attacks. However, fear was not a part of a primordials' character so he did not brood over it in that manner. Nonetheless, another characteristic of a primordial was to always let it be known that they were to be respected and honored.

Those plotting against him had apparently forgotten such things and would have to be taught a lesson. As much as Rah hated having to make others suffer, he also could not allow anyone to think that he was not to be respected. Thus, he would have to proceed with his plans to reinstate order, justice and harmony in that regard.

# Eight

Centuries had passed and Afro-dite grew tired of being alone. Besides that she had created even more powers and perfected them all to the point of boredom. So she decided that it was time to return to Sirius and thought herself back there.

When she arrived she felt that something was off, but couldn't quite put her finger on what it was. She wasn't ready to face her father right away so the first person that she went to see was her mother to get a feel for how her father was doing.

"Oh my Afro-dite you're back!" Amaunet said running up to hug her daughter showering her with kisses. "Where have you been? Your father has been sick with worry over you. You really hurt him taking off like that. He's not doing too well you know," Amaunet said as she welcomed Afro-dite back home.

"Dad is sick? Oh no what's wrong with him mom? I didn't mean to worry you. I didn't think I'd been gone that long," Afro-dite replied.

"You didn't need to be gone long. It's the way you took off. How could you leave like that in the middle of your birthday party? Your father was devastated after that," Amaunet explained.

Hearing that her father was ill made Afro-dite feel horrible for having run off the way that she had. She knew how her father was with her. He was very protective of her. So when she ran off she should have known that it would gravely affect him.

"I'm sorry mom. I didn't mean for all of that to happen. I just needed some time to think. Where is dad? Is he here?," Afro-dite inquired beginning to feel a pang of guilt shoot through her heart.

She loved her father more than existence itself and she felt awful for having caused him so much pain. She needed to see him right away to try to smooth things over and get him back to better health. She knew that just seeing her would instantly heal him. It was his heart that needed to be healed and that was making him sick. She had broken his heart and she knew that she needed to mend it.

"He may be in our room. He went out earlier, but I think he may be back by now. You should go and see him right away," Amaunet instructed.

"I will mom. I'm sorry for running off like that and hurting you both that way. It was very selfish of me. I don't know what I was thinking. I'd better go and see dad," Afro-dite said apologetically.

With that Afto-dite took off to go and see

about her father.

# Nine

When Afro-dite arrived in the room it was just as her mother had described. Her father looked very ill. He seemed to have aged 30 megaannum. Upon the sight of him, overcome with worry, Afro-dite ran over to her father and hugged him tightly.

"You've come home! You've returned sunshine!" Rah gleamed.

"Yes dad. I'm sorry that I ran off like that. I shouldn't have. I guess you were right and that I'm not mature enough to go on a mission. That was very childish of me to run off like that. I do hope that you'll forgive me. You were right dad," Afro-dite said beginning to pout.

"Oh sunshine don't cry and there is nothing to forgive. I'm the one that needs your forgiveness. I should have believed in you. I could have given you a chance. You were right. I'm just glad you're back. Will you ever forgive me?" Rah asked his daughter who couldn't believe what she was hearing.

"Yes dad, yes! So you *do* believe in me even though I acted so immature running off the way I did?" Afro-dite asked.

"Of course I believe in you. I have always believed in you sunshine. It was never lack of belief that kept me from sending you on a mission. It was my concern for your safety. There are many who want to see me fall and who want desperately to take my place and so I never wanted to run the risk of them coming after you to try to get to me. Being out there isn't all fun and action dear. There is much danger that I have gone out of my way to shield you from," Rah explained.

"Yeah dad, but I too have great powers, greater than even *you* know about. I've been perfecting them for some time and I'm really good," Afro-dite revealed anxious to see her father's response.

"Oh yeah is that so. Hmmmm…. Show me these powers dear," Rah commanded.

Then, looking as though his words were music to her ears Afro-dite promptly honored her father's wishes and showed her father her new powers. She also revealed to him all the time that she spent in the Majestic Forest creating, developing and perfecting her new powers and describing to him all that they could do. To her surprise Rah was impressed.

"Wow sunshine! I had no idea. You *have* been working. Why did you keep this a secret from me? We have always shared everything," Rah asked.

"I didn't feel like you'd be okay with it.

Besides that I wanted to make sure I had it together when I came to you. I know you want me to stay your little girl dad, but I'm growing up now and you've always raised me for greatness. After all I *am* the daughter of Rah, the greatest of all creators. So I wanted to wait until I could skillfully represent that greatness. But when I was ready and you denied me the chance to show you I just got really upset," Afro-dite explained.

"I understand dear one and I'm sorry that I made you feel that you couldn't come to me before. However, now that I know what you can do I actually have a mission for you and it's a very important one," Rah replied.

Afro-dite couldn't believe her ears. What she had just heard was what she'd waited for her entire life and it was music to her ears. She felt like she was in a dream and for a moment she thought that she might have been.

Being assigned a mission from Rah was

a great honor for anyone. It wasn't the sort of thing to be taken lightly and it said a lot about his level of trust in Afro-dite so she was excited to hear more.

# Ten

Overcome with joy Afro-dite listened on. She couldn't believe that her dream was finally coming true. Her father was not only sending her on a mission, but it was an important, top secret one.

Rah shared with her all that he knew of some of the titans and gods trying to overthrow him. He told her even more than Amaunet had informed her of earlier. He explained to her that he didn't trust anyone, especially those closest to him.

"Dad are you saying that think that mom might be in on this?" Afro-dite asked.

"Oh never! Amaunet would never do such a thing. We are bound together as one so for her to do that would be the same as doing that to herself. Besides that her love and yours are the only love that I know to be real," Rah replied.

"I'm just saying that it's possibly one among the primordial beings who may be in on it. I don't want to think that but you never know with these things. However, I doubt that is so, but I'm just taking all the precautions to make sure," Rah added.

Afro-dite couldn't believe her ears. Everyone had always had the utmost respect for her father so the thought that they had turned on him made her angry. After all Rah had done so much for them. In fact, if it weren't for Rah they wouldn't even exist as he was their creator.

Rah was the father of all creation. Thus, they all owed their existence to him. Besides that he had never done anything but love any of them. Even when they defied him he loved them nonetheless.

The more Afro-dite listened the angrier she became. Afro-dite couldn't wait to leave for the mission. She was more ready to take them all out if necessary. As far as she was concerned her powers far exceeded all of their combined and so she was ready for battle.

As Rah looked as his maturing daughter he had all the faith in the world in her. So without further hesitation he gave her all of the details of the mission and got her prepared to go.

He told her what to look for, where to begin looking. He also told her how to go undercover and how to avoid compromising her cover. He told her what dangers to look out for and avoid as well as what he considered the most important rule, which was to never quit the mission. Afro-dite soaked it all in like a sponge.

Since the mission was top secret and no one other than the two of them knew of the details they decided that her departure would be done in secret as well at the Rah hour, which was the hour of sunrise. They planned to use the brightness of the sun, which no being could see beyond, as her disguise. So as planned that next day Afro-dite left for her first mission.

# Eleven

Afro-dite's arrival on planet Earth was all that she thought it would be. The trip there went smoothly and as she parted ways with Rah she saw in his eyes the look of a father's pride that she always dreamt of seeing. It was all that she needed to give her the confidence necessary to successfully complete her first mission.

The year on Earth was 2028 and Afro-dite had arrived in a city called New York. She entered the city in secret, arising from what was called the Hudson River by way of her grandfather, Nun. Having taken on human form Afro-dite arrived as an 11 year old girl as was what she and her father agreed would be best.

For the most part she was fairly average

looking. She maintained only a fraction of her natural primordial beauty. However, she still had much of her beautiful hair. It was just a lot more toned down than in it's original form. She had brown piercing eyes and was a caramel brown complexion.

What she did maintain of her primordial self was her powers. Rah told her that though it risked blowing her cover she had to keep her powers even in physical form because she would need them to carry out the mission.

Essentially, Afro-dite looked average enough to blend in. No one knew of her powers and she planned to never use them openly. Doing so would ensure that her cover wouldn't be blown.

She did everything that she could to be almost invisible. Blending in was her top priority. She didn't need all of the attention that coming to Earth as a goddess would bring as that would have been too much of a distraction and would make her prey to too many dangers. She didn't know who among the humans was after her father so she had to maintain a low profile.

# Twelve

Afro-dite was so excited about getting started. Though she'd heard all about how sneaky and underhanded humans could be she was still very much looking forward to getting in the mix and seeing who they were for herself. Besides that she was anxious to see who among them was plotting against her father.

The first part of her mission was to come up with a good cover. She had to blend in and give no one so much as a hint as to who she was. So the first thing that she did, blending in with her child's body to remain invisible, was study humanity.

She studied every aspect of humanity from their submission to their emotions to their disdain for one another. She couldn't understand why one set of humans so disliked another set of humans or why there were even separated into sets to begin with.

She also couldn't understand why the darker ones among them were so hated. It seemed the entire planet conspired against them. The darker ones had been enslaved, taken advantage of, deceived and rejected by the other sets. Then within the set of darker ones there was even more hatred among them.

The lighter ones didn't like the darker ones and vice versa. Then the educated ones didn't like the uneducated ones. The ones with money didn't like the ones without money. The religious didn't like the non-religious and one religious set didn't like another. The straight-haired ones didn't like the curly-haired ones and it seemed the list of divisions among them just seemed to go on and on.

Afro-dite was totally confused by all the chaos that existed amongst the humans and despite all of her attempts to make sense of and understand it she found that in doing so she became that much more confused.

Nonetheless, she was sent to complete a mission so she made it her business to stay focused on doing just that.  The last thing that she was going to do was get caught up in all the human drama because dramatic they were!

It wasn't hard for Afro-dite to establish a cover.  She got herself adopted by a family who lived in what was called the southeast side of Queens in a town called Hollis.  Before she arrived Rah had used his power of implanting memories to make the family believe Afro-dite to be the daughter of a cousin who had died of illness.

The family was made to believe that since no other family member stepped up to adopt the child they were to offer to do it.  So obediently, upon Afro-dite's arrival, they took her into their home.  Rah took great care in selecting this particular family as he wanted his daughter cared for in a loving home.

Warm and loving they were as they fell in love with Afro-dite the instant they saw her as did most. Even in mortal form she was a vision of pure beauty that radiated far beyond the physical eyes.

Her adopted parents were also very impressed with Afro-dite's ability to speak several languages and her intelligence. They believed that she spoke 3 languages fluently including English, Spanish and French as she had communicated with several of the neighbors fluent in those languages.

What they didn't realize was that in being a primordial, Afro-dite could communicate with all beings and in all languages. So language was not a barrier for her as it seemed to be for the humans. She discovered that different sets of humans spoke different languages, which other sets often did not understand. For Afro-dite, that was just yet another thing on the already long list of things that kept the humans divided.

The more time she spent among the humans the more she learned of their division. In her opinion, it was the cause of their weakness.

Afro-dite studied every aspect of the humans from their frailties to their common desires. As for their common desires, what she noticed was that no matter what set of humans she studied they all seemed to have a strong desire to be happy and feel love.

However, what confused her was that while they all shared this admirable desire it seemed that it was also those same desires that was the source of their weakness as humans. Humans seemed to do some of the most hateful things to one another to feel happy about themselves and all in the name of love.

They bullied, hated and treated others

badly to make themselves feel happy about themselves. They hurt one another and said they did it because they loved them. They did dangerous things that risked their very existence like jump out of planes saying that it made them feel happy and free. They knowingly ate the very foods that they knew made them sick saying that the food made them happy. Afro-dite found that there was a long list of similar contradictions that was as long as the list of divisions. In fact, there were so many contradictions that Afro-dite almost got lost in them.

Humanity was as usual too overwhelming for Afro-dite to get distracted with. So she decided to again focus back on the mission. She had to figure out a way to locate those who were out to get her father.

After some observation she had come up with the perfect plan and had figured out exactly where she would start. It wasn't the most obvious, but it was a good plan. She decided to use her hair as her ticket in.

# Thirteen

Hair was something that Afro-dite knew to be very powerful among the humans. At the same time, it happened to also be the source of Afro-dite's power. In the heavens it was well-known that hair was like an antenna. In many cases it was a gateway of sorts.

This was not something that was known or understood by the human species as the frequency that they were tuned into was not one that would allow them to have awareness of such knowledge. Yet, those among the more highly evolved knew very well of such high sciences.

So Afro-dite knew that by using hair as a means of tracking who among the humans had awareness of such high sciences she could zero in on the identity of those who were conspiring against her father. As she began to focus more and more on identifying the conspirators at times Afro-dite became more and disturbed. The humans, the gods, the titans all angered her. Them and lack of gratitude for all that Rah had done for them. She was utterly shocked by their lack of gratitude and often thought to herself, "The nerve of them!"

Nonetheless, even those thoughts were distractions and taking Afro-dite off track so she kept her cool about such things and stayed focused. She knew that when she located the traitors they would know well of her wrath. So she like the predator that she was planned to quietly sit, wait, stalk and strategically map out her attack.

A few days had passed when after using her powers of magnetism Afro-dite drew to her the first bread crumb on the path to locating her father's traitors. It was the beginning of Afro-dite's 6th grade year in middle school and she the first bread crumb came in the form of a confrontation that she had with some children from the neighborhood.

Afro-dite was walking home from school when one of the girls from school said, "Well if it ain't the black orphan Annie and she even has the nappy afro too," while laughing as some other children joined in.

"Girl you need to tame that wild kingdom on your head," teased another.

"Yeah! Did you just come from time traveling? Cause girl that hairstyle went out about a hundred years ago. Want us to take you to the hairdresser and get that thing updated?" taunted another.

Afro-dite listened on in amusement. She wasn't at all offended by the mockery as she did not see it as such. To her the children's fascination with her hair was a compliment and let her know things were all going according to plan.

She actually even thought that some of what they said about her hair was flattering.  It was particularly the part about going to the hairdresser.  She had no idea that hair could get dressed up.  She couldn't wait to get that done to hers.

She also didn't know that children from Earth knew how to time travel.  She had always been told that they were very primitive and didn't know about such things.  She started to think that perhaps humans weren't so bad and for a moment she began to enjoy being on Earth and even entertained the prospect of staying for a while.

However, the fondness that Afro-dite was developing for the humans was short-lived after what happened next.  While the other children were launching verbal attacks one very bold girl decided to grab and yank out a lock of Afro-dite's hair.  Then, the little girl extended the hair out seeing it's length and said that she was going to cut all of Afro-dite's hair off and use it to make hair weave.

Afro-dite had not yet been introduced to hair weave. She's seen it, but never knew that's what it was. She would use her power of energy reading on those around her who wore hair weaves to try to get a better idea of what it was about.

However, what she'd notice was that something was very off with it. Yet, she couldn't identify exactly what it was. So the hair weave became the unsolved mystery that Afro-dite was itching to solve. So she wasn't sure what the girls that wore hair weaves had on their head. From what she read from it's energy whatever it was had been something that she had never before seen.

So when the little girl made reference to a hair weave Afro-dite wondered if the thing called a weave was what was responsible for the strange energy flowing from many of the girls' heads.

For Afro-dite this was a clue in the right direction and so she made it a point to investigate it further. In the meantime, she had to immediately address the matter of the child who yanked out a loc of her hair and threatened to cut the rest. Afro-dite not only had to address it, but she had to ensure that the others knew better than try it again in the future.

# Fourteen

Afro-dite's hair was sacred and more than that it was in great part the source of her newly gained powers, specifically the ones that she developed on her own. When she developed the powers of healing and command over the elements on her own she did so by binding both powers to her hair.

Thus, anyone making threats against her hair did so at their own risk, including the little girl. Besides that each strand of Afro-dite's hair was a living entity, which she considered her child. So her response to attacks and threats against her hair were pretty serious, to say the least.

Immediately after the little girl had snatched out the lock of Afro-dite's hair she instantly felt a sharp pain in her chest. For a moment her heart sank as she briefly mourned the death of what she considered one of her beloved children who had died from the separation. The grief instantly transformed to anger making Afro-dite raging mad like a wild bull!

Knowing how dangerous it could become for the humans if her rage reached its full capacity Afro-dite quickly snapped out of it invoking all of her willpower to do so. She had to try her best to avoid striking out at the girl as she knew that doing so would be the death of the child. After all, she was a primordial being and the little girl was a mere human so the fight would have been no contest.

Nonetheless, Afro-dite was a very caring mother to her creations. She was driven to protect them at all cost and that time was no exception. So the only thing that kept her from striking out at the little girl was that when she did an energy scan on the child she saw that around her was a dark, murky pink color.

For Afro-dite energy scan revealed the truth about a person.  It showed up as different colors.  The dark, murky pink color that was around the little girl meant that she was just immature and pretending to be tough to save face with the other children.  This made Afro-dite actually feel sorry for the little girl as she knew it to be yet another common weakness that many humans suffered from.

During her time on Earth Afro-dite had found that immaturity and dishonesty were very common traits among human.  They were always trying to hide their true selves from one another.  Yet despite their ability to deceive one another energy never lied.  So Afro-dite began to dismiss such flaws as something that she really didn't need to be concerned with.

That being the case she gave the little girl a pass and didn't strike her down.  Instead she invoked her power of command over the elements and sent the wind to pick up a nearby piece of garbage that was lying on the ground and smacked the girl in the face with it.

The swift smack against her cheek sounded almost like a hand smack and sent the other children into a fit of laughter. This made the little girl embarrassed so she went sulking away holding her head down in shame.

It was the punishment that Afro-dite thought was well deserved. She considered the little girl very lucky as she was for the most part one of the most compassionate and loving among primordials, gods, humans and other beings alike.

Though, like everything else in the universe there was another side of Afro-dite that was quite the opposite of loving that could strike out anytime she was provoked. It was the side of Afro-dite that her father's traitors would soon know.

# Fifteen

As the days went on and the more time she spent with them the more Afro-dite found that the children had quite a fascination with teasing her about her hair. It was weird to Afro-dite that they would tease her about such a thing because where she was from her hair was always her most liked quality. However, the children in the Earthly realm seemed to view her hair as just the opposite. They would tease her about it daily.

Most days, Afro-dite wore her hair in a huge afro. It was thick, tightly coiled and a lot dryer than she was used to. It seemed the air in the Earthly realm soaked up all of it's natural oils, which made it appear very dry and a lot more difficult to manage.

In fact, her adopted mother, Jackie, would struggle with it everyday. No matter what Jackie tried, it seemed that Afro-dite's hair just didn't want to be managed and as a result it gave Jackie the hardest time.

It fought her, it mocked her, it challenged her and eventually it wore Jackie down. When Jackie tried to make Afro-dite's hair lay down, like a coil wire it popped right back up. When Jackie tried to make Afro-dite's hair straight and smooth it became curly and frizzy bush. When Jackie tried to make Afro-dite's hair shine the roots would soak up all the oils like a starving dessert leaving the rest dry and brittle.

It didn't matter what Jackie did Afro-dite's hair would stand it's ground. Jackie began to see Afro-dite's hair as something that she was at war with. She bought all types of weapons to fight against it from combs and brushes to straightening combs, barrettes, bows, hair grease mixtures and all of the proclaimed latest and greatest in shampoos and conditioners.

Afro-dite's hair was just too much like her and it insisted on doing whatever it wanted. Then because she was the daughter of Rah everyone had always allowed her do just that. Though, on Earth things were very different as Afro-dite would soon find out.

Not having ever had any type of comb put on her hair, one day Jackie tried to straighten Afro-dite's hair with a straightening comb. Lo and behold when she laid the piping hot comb on Afro-dite's hair the deafening screams of a million souls rang out in Afro-dite's ears and she felt a sharp pain in the very depths of her soul. The comb, like an atomic bomb sent explosions into the coils of her hair as Afro-dite's hair screamed out in agonizing pain.

Afro-dite thought to herself, "What is this weapon of mass destruction being raked through my hair?"

Then, as if by way of an automatic reflex, Afro-dite used her powers to strike out against Jackie causing the comb to instantly snap in half. Afro-dite didn't do it on purpose, but protecting her hair was like an automatic response.

Jackie couldn't believe her eyes. She'd never seen anything like that happen in all of her years of combing hair. She had two girls of her own, Candi who was 15 and Carla who was 8, whose hair she hot combed all the time. Yet, never once had she ever seen a thick, metal, wide-toothed straightening comb break in half.

Knowing what she'd done Afro-dite looked at the metal comb and smiled. She didn't know what the gadget was or why it was being used to attack her hair, but from that day forward she kept her defenses up against it.

Jackie ended up buying and breaking 2 more straightening combs before she finally gave in.

The more time she spent on Earth, the more Afro-dite saw the need to keep her hair's defenses up. It was like an endless war zone. It seemed there was always some evil force coming for her hair. If it wasn't children attacking her hair it was hot combs, plastic combs, blow dryers, hard brushes, shampoos, chemical liquids and a long list of other threats. She was finding it more and more difficult to focus on the mission at hand with having to constantly stop to protect her hair.

Nonetheless, after the incident with Jackie she made it her business to stay focused on the mission at all cost. She had to do some investigating into what the weave was and what it was doing to the girls and women on Earth.

She had a feeling that it all had something to do with who was after her father.

So she began to focus her efforts on getting to the bottom of it. Time was running out and she didn't know when the traitor would strike. Though she had a feeling that it would be sooner rather than later.

# Sixteen

The next day, Afro-dite decided to ask her cousin, Candi about weave. Candi was Jackie's 15-year-old daughter who often wore the same weaves that were giving off the strange energy that Afro-dite had been noticing on many of the girls at school.

It was a Saturday morning so everyone was at home. They lived in a small, 2-bedroom apartment on 191st Street and Woodhull Ave. The apartment was nothing fancy, but Jackie kept it fairly clean.

Upon first entering the apartment there was a large living room combined with a dining room. In the living room there was a large black leather couch and matching love seat. In the center of the room was a large television set that sat on a glass tv stand. In the dining room was a square wooden table that seated up to six people.

Then off to the right of the living room was a small kitchen. The kitchen was kept very clean and was usually the cleanest kept room in the apartment.

Back towards the rear of the apartment were two bedrooms and a bathroom. The largest room was called the master bedroom. In the master bedroom was a queen-sized bed dressed in brown bedsheets and a spread. There were also two dressers and two nightstands. The furniture was all black lacquer and seemed rather old.

In the other bedroom was a bunk bed set. The bottom bed, where Candi and Carla slept, was a full-sized bed dressed in mint green bed sheets and a comforter. The top bunk, where Afro-dite slept, was a twin-sized bed dressed in the same bedding as the bottom bunk. There was also a white wooden vertical-standing, 3-drawer dresser, which had one drawer for each girl.

Jackie's husband Alan worked all the time so it seemed they rarely saw him except for Saturday and Sunday mornings and that was only if he wasn't working overtime. He worked for the New York City Transit Authority, better known as the TA. Alan had worked there for over 20 years.

Afro-dite was very fascinated with how dedicated humans were to working though it was a concept that she really didn't quite understood. She couldn't understand why humans worked day in and day out spending so much of their time doing tedious tasks that had nothing to do with their evolution.

In Sirius and many other worlds it was all about evolving and gaining more knowledge, wisdom and understanding. Doing so helped one move up to the next, more evolved dimension or reality, which was like moving to a better world where they had more powers.  So everyone spent all of their time working on themselves, learning more and fixing their imperfections.

It was very different from Earth where everyone seemed to waste entire lifetimes doing things that didn't at all improve their race.

Afro-dite would hear them say that they worked to pay bills, yet the bills that they had didn't make any sense to Afro-dite either.  She thought to herself that it made no sense for them to pay for things like shelter, land, gas, water, electric, food or any of the other things humans said were necessary when her father provided all of those things to them for free.  To her knowledge he had never charged what the humans call money for anything.

The more she observed the state of affairs on Earth the more she began to suspect that something major was happening and therefore she needed to find out exactly what that was. Eventually, she chalked the whole going to work and money thing that humans were so obsessed with up to being yet another of their flaws that would likely never make any sense.

# Seventeen

As Afro-dite watched Candi get ready she thought to herself that someone was using the humans to get to Rah and she had to find out who that was and she needed to start with the weave clue. So while Candi was ironing her clothes to go out somewhere Afro-dite decided to talk to her about it.

"Hi Candi! You heading out?" Afro-dite asked.

"Yeah, I'm going out with some friends later to the movies and I just want to get my clothes ironed now. But first, I need to go by the beauty supply store after I iron my clothes so that Angie can do my hair," Candi replied.

Angie was her best friend who came by the apartment quite a bit to see Candi and hang out.  She lived in the same apartment building on a different floor so she was always coming over.

"Oh, the beauty supply store!  What's that?" Afro-dite asked.

Looking at her strangely Candi replied, "It's just a store where you buy stuff for your hair and nails.  I need to pick up some hair. You want to come?" Candi asked.

"Yeah!  I'd love to!" Afro-dite gleamed excited about learning more about the hair fascination.  "But why do you have to *buy* hair? Isn't that hair on your head and isn't it free?" Afro-dite asked curiously.

Laughing Candi answered, "Yeah I do have hair and it is free, but I like to wear different hairstyles.  Somedays I like my hair short, some days long and somedays I like different colors.  Today I want to wear it long so that's why I'm going to pick up some hair."

"Fascinating," Afro-dite thought to herself.  She couldn't wait to learn more and see what the beauty supply store was like.  She never needed supplies for beauty as she was known as one of the most beautiful beings in existence.

The weird things that humans did simply amazed Afro-dite.  They worked day in and day out to pay for things that the Earth produced free.  Meanwhile, they also wanted money to pay for other things like beauty.  Human nature was intriguing.

Thus, Afro-dite was filled with excitement at the prospect of learning more.  So she went to get dressed to go out with Candi and do just that.

As Afro-dite watched Candi get dressed she realized that she too needed to get dressed as well.  She would have worn what she had on, but when she'd done so previously she was scolded and told that it was not appropriate to go 'out' in pajamas.

For Afro-dite the humans just had too many hang-ups and way too many rules. In Sirius there were only seven, but on Earth the list was endless. There was no wonder why their existence was so riddled with confusion and why they weren't as highly evolved as other beings throughout the universe.

# Eighteen

About a half an hour later Afro-dite and Candi had arrived at the Paradise Beauty Supply store. It was about 12 blocks away from the apartment so they walked. Twelve blocks was considered rather a short distance to the humans in New York who seemed to walk everywhere. It seemed rather long to Afro-dite who was used to teleporting so it was something that she had to get used to.

When they arrived at the beauty supply store Afro-dite was amazed at all the hair weaves and wigs there were to choose from. They had some that were kinky, some that were straight and some that were curly. They also came in different colors. So they had some that were blonde, some that were black and some that were red and brown.

Then for the weaves there two types which were called synthetic and human hair. Human hair seemed to be the most popular. Afro-dite couldn't believe that it actually came from the heads of humans. She looked around in awe.

As she looked around she realized that the decision-making process took a long time. It seemed they were in the store for hours. Candi wanted to see one sample after another. Each time she'd run her fingers through it, hold it up to her had and look at it in the mirror. Then she changed her mind several times as to which color she wanted. At first she wanted brown, then she wanted red and then she went back to brown. Once she finally made a decision as to color she couldn't decide whether she wanted curly or straight hair.

Then at last, after what seemed like an eternity Candi decided on a straight, light brown pack of human hair. Her natural hair was a dark brown and about ear length so she had planned to extend the length of hair to about midway down her back.

Then, as they headed to the counter Afro-dite saw something that struck her as odd. The woman who rang Candi up at the cash register had a strange energy field. She was a short, stocky, middle aged black woman with shoulder length sandy brown hair. What was strange about her was that though she read as human, she did not read as a typical human.

Yet, when Afro-dite looked at the lady more closely the woman didn't even read as human at all. In fact, there was something very off about her energy field altogether that caught Afro-dite completely off guard.

Afro-dite blinked unable to believe her human eyes. She recognized the woman's energy field as being that of a highly evolved being! Afro-dite couldn't believe it!

To her knowledge she was the only highly evolved entity on the planet at the time. More than that no one else was permitted to be there without her father's permission and to her knowledge Rah had not granted anyone but her permission to be there.

Calmly and so as not to alert the woman that Afro-dite recognized her, Afro-dite studied the woman's movements trying to figure out who she was. She figured that it had to be one of the gods in disguise because no one else was strong enough to break past the quarantine.

Some time previously Rah had quarantined the planet in order to protect the humans. Because humans were on the low end of evolution they were vulnerable. So the quarantine kept other highly evolved beings who were a lot stronger and powerful from taking advantage of humans. It also kept humanity from being distracted and focused on their own evolution.

So for there to be another highly evolved being on the planet besides Afro-dite meant that whoever else was on Earth had to be there with less than good intentions. Seeing the woman Afro-dite knew that she was getting very close to figuring out who was trying to take down her dad.

Meanwhile, Afro-dite kept her cool and maintained her cover so that the lady, or whoever she was, didn't recognize her. Prior to coming to the planet Afro-dite had created an energetic cloak that kept her true identity undetectable. So she was pretty sure that no one would recognize her. Nonetheless, she still made sure that she blended in.

Candi paid for her hair and the two of them headed for the door. Then just as they were heading out the door in walked one of the little girls who often teased Afro-dite. She was with another little girl who Afro-dite had never seen. They all looked at one another in passing without saying a word. Then Afro-dite followed the little girl with her eyes and saw that she went to say something to the woman at the register.

"Are those some of your friends from school A?" Candi inquired.

"No not a friend, but she does go to my school," Afro-dite answered blankly.

"Oh. Have you made any friends at school yet?" Candi prodded.

"No, not really," Afro-dite answered.

"Oh no. Well maybe I can help. Some of my friends have little sisters that go there that are about your age," Candi offered.

Afro-dite did not respond as she was too deep in thought about what had just happened in the store. Afro-dite was happy to finally have a lead on who was out to get Rah. She at least knew where to look for the next clue. So from that day forward she stayed very alert. It wasn't long before she found another clue.

# Nineteen

Later that day Angie came over to put the weave in Candi's hair.

"Hi Ms. Jackie!  I'm just here to help Candi do something with her hair," Angie greeted sweeping through the door as was her normal way of entering.

"Good.  Come on in.  I'm glad you're here cause that girl needs something done to that nest," Jackie replied making her way back to the couch was she was sitting before opening the door for Angie.

Laughing Angie replied, "Now Ms. Jackie you know you ain't right.  She's been keeping her hair up pretty good lately.  At least she's keeping it touched up now."

"Yeah speaking of which do you think you can do something to that one's hair?" Jackie said said pointing to Afro-dite who was sitting on the floor reading a book.

"Whew now that's a lot right there. I don't know about that Ms. Jackie. I wouldn't know where to start. It's just too much. What are you doing with it now? Have you thought about perming it?" Angie inquired.

"I sure want to, but she won't let anyone come near it. I tried to straighten it with the hot comb and girl do you know the comb broke in half!?!?!! Three of them!!!" Jackie exclaimed.

"What! Ms. Jackie you're kidding. Whose hair can break a metal straightening comb! Wow, you're gonna have to do something about that. That's a serious problem. So are you gonna perm it?" Angie asked again.

"No I still think she's too young for that,

but I was thinking about getting it braided. At least then it would last for a while and I could get somewhat of a break. Don't you braid too?" Jackie asked Angie.

"Yeah that might be a good idea. I could definitely braid it, but I gotta tell you Ms. Jackie that with all that hair she got I'm gonna have to charge you," Angie replied.

"Girl that is not a problem. I will gladly pay you to take that nightmare off my hands. So I'll have Candi pick up the hair and then let you know. I would definitely appreciate that cause that nest looks like a project gone wrong. That's a lot of hair right there and it's so thick. There's no way I need to be trying to tackle that everyday! Then she won't let nobody come near it. I guess she's bracing herself," Jackie explained.

"Yeah well with hair that thick I'd be tensing up too. She's probably used to it hurting. I'm gonna have to bring lots of moisturizer when I do her hair," Angie added.

While Jackie and Angie continued discussing Afro-dite's hair as if she wasn't even sitting there Candi had joined them in the livingroom. She had been in the girls room trying to tidy up before Angie got there.

They usually did Candi's hair back in the girl's room, which was kind of a mess from Candi's younger sister, Carla playing with all of her dolls earlier. When Candi came out Angie began gathering her hair dressing materials to head back to the room.

"Hey girl! You ready?" Angie asked before pausing and looking at Candi's hair dramatically. "Whew look at that! Yes you're ready! Well at least this time it's touched up so I don't have to work as hard," Angie fussed as they headed back to the room.

Afro-dite sat brewing over all that was just discussed. She was still surprised about what humans thought about their hair, particularly black ones. It seemed to them hair was the center of everything.

They invested a lot of time, money and conversation on hair. Then there was the obsession over the different types of hair that didn't even belong to black people that they seemed obsessed with wearing.

When Afro-dite went to the beauty supply store she learned that black women particularly liked to wear 5 types of hair which included Brazilian, Peruvian, Indian, Malaysian and Eurasian. This confused her more than ever. For the life of her she couldn't understand why the black women didn't like their own hair type.

It was free, it was strong, it was curly, it was unique and it was beautiful. So going to the beauty supply store to buy hair that didn't at all match their own hair type under the guise of doing so to make themselves beautiful made no sense to Afro-dite.  The more time she spent learning about black hair the more Afro-dite began to suspect that it was all tied to her mission.  She was even more than convinced of this when she saw Candi's hair.

Enjoying this book so far? I'd love for you to share your thoughts and post a quick review on Amazon!

# Twenty

When Angie was done with Candi's hair Afro-dite noticed the strangest thing.  Candi's energy field looked just like the lady in the beauty supply store.

She looked again and when she did Afro-dite was positive that Candi's energy field was human before getting the weave as she had been with her all day.  However, something had definitely changed.

Immediately, Afro-dite grabbed a piece of the hair.  She knew that the energy shift had to be linked to the weave so she wanted to prove her hunch.  She picked up the strands of hair weave, which Candi called 'Brazilian human hair.'  Afro-dite then used her command over the elements to separate the elements out of the human hair in order to get to the root of what was foreign in the hair. She found that there was oxygen, carbon, hydrogen, nitrogen and sulphur, none of which was a surprise as they were commonly found in all human hair.

However, what she also found was that there was a foreign element that was causing her to get a non-human read from the energy field. She had to look twice because she couldn't believe what she was seeing!

Seeing how strangely Afro-dite was looking at her, Candi asked, "You like it 'A?' It's pretty right?"

"Oh yeah, it's really nice," Afro-dite answered. Then to break the awkward silence she asked, "So your hair is still there?"

"Yes, it's just braided underneath," Candi answered as she made her way to the kitchen to get a snack. "Angie, did you want a snack?"

Candi asked turning her attention to Angie.

"No thank you. I need to go get dressed. I'll be back up when it's time to go," Angie said heading out the door.

"Ok see you later," Candi yelled behind her.

Since Jackie had gone to the store, Carla was taking a nap and Candi was getting dressed to head out Afro-dite decided to take a few minutes to put some things together for her mission. She typically worked on such things at night, but since she'd made so much progress that day she figured it was okay to do a little work during the day.

Afro-dite still had the strands of hair from Candi's weave and she wanted to examine it again. It definitely had clues in it that she needed to identify. So taking a moment to take a closer look Afro-dite saw something that she hadn't gotten a chance to see before.

The hair had an energy grid that was identical to the earth's energy grid. Afro-dite could not believe her eyes! Yet, it all made sense. She had figured it out!

The humans were not a part of trying to take Rah out! In fact, they were being used by the real culprit who behind the whole scheme and who was actually channeling energy from the humans to give them the power needed to take Rah out. So they were essentially using the humans as batteries. Afro-dite couldn't believe how close she was getting to identifying who that was.

She was really beginning to piece a lot of things together. The earth's energy grid was like electrical strings that connected at points, which were called power centers. Each power center had surges of power. So all over the Earth were these power centers, which had gushes of power coming from the. It was almost like having several small suns on certain spots on the earth.

Yet, the most interesting thing about all of this was that the hair weaves had an identical energy grid as the planet Earth. What this told Afro-dite about hair weaves was that someone was using women who wore hair weaves to create energy grids that were being channeled to build up their own power. It was a genius plan and it all made sense!

The human brain generated between 10 to 23 watts of power a day. The energy generated from the human brain paired with the power spots of the energy grid that Afro-dite saw in the hair strands on the hair weave would be like a mega power surge that could shake the whole of existence.

This all blew Afro-dite's mind! She *had* to get to the bottom of who was behind this. Even more importantly she had to figure out what they were planning. She knew that she would need to harness as much of her powers as possible because she was certainly going to need it to go up against whoever was behind all of this.

The more Afro-dite thought about it all she couldn't believe her luck!  She never imagined that her first mission would be such an important one.  Her father's faith in her was proven beyond a doubt.  Though the pressure was on Afro-dite was so thrilled that Rah had given her such an important job.

Yet, Afro-dite's excitement was short-lived.  Things began to unfold a lot faster than she was ready for.  So sooner than expected her excitement turned to anxiety as Afro-dite felt the pressure of needing to plan and act quickly.  It was all the unknown for her, but she wouldn't get any second chances so she had to be ready for anything.

Afro-dite spent the remainder of the evening planning what to do next.  She also spent time working out in her head the possibilities of who could be behind the whole scheme.  Time was definitely of the essence.

# Twenty-One

Later that same night as was always the case Afro-dite went to work on identifying the traitor.   She still suspected that the lady at the beauty supply store had something to do with it. There was just something about her.

So all that night Afro-dite was deep in thought.  As a primordial being she didn't sleep. Though to maintain her cover she *pretended* to sleep every night, which wasn't too difficult to do from the top bunk.   So every night she closed her eyes, but sleep she did not.  What she did instead was shift her consciousness to other planes of existence.  She did this so that she could continue her work.

There were several planes of existence. Like the physical plane that the humans existed on, there were several others that other beings existed on and that more highly evolved beings were able to shift between at will.

That night Afro-dite shifted to what was known as the primordial plane to check in with her father. After learning what she had learned earlier that day she absolutely had to give him an update.

It didn't take long for Afro-dite to shift back to the primordial plans as she was more than happy to be back. Though the more time she spent in human form the more difficult it was at times to shift back because the human body was solid and heavy. Shifting to the higher realms required that one be light as those realms were light. Thus, for Afro-dite it essentially meant that in order to shift she had to become less human and doing so became increasingly more difficult.

Afro-dite went through great pains to keep her humanity to a minimum so as not to lose her primordial self in her temporary human experience. In fact, one way that she did that was through her nightly shifts back to her primordial form. So her nighttime activities became somewhat of a job.

# Twenty-Two

That night she had to completely shift so that she could speak to her father. She closed her eyes and within a few minutes she was back at Sirius.

She didn't want to risk anyone else seeing her so she appeared to her father as a dream. Running up to hug him she said, "Dad I'm so glad to see you. I've missed you so much! Being down there is really lonely."

"I know but it is only for a short while. You will be back home before you know it. How is my sunshine? You have come to tell me what you have learned?" Rah asked.

"Yes dad I have. There is someone very highly evolved who has betrayed you.

You are correct in taking so many precautions and maintaining secrecy. Please do not share my mission to anyone, not even those closest to you. Dad I fear that it may be someone greatly trusted by the family who is behind this. Whoever, came up with this plan is highly intelligent and has worked on this for millions of years. That means they know everything about you," Afro-dite informed.

"Well that can't be so because no one in existence knows everything about me, not even you, not even your mother. They may know a great deal about me, but I assure you they don't know everything. So are you close to identifying the traitor?" Rah asked.

"I am very close dad. I just came to warn you to maintain a very watchful eye on all of those within reach of you. From what I have learned they are trying to be even more powerful than you," Afro-dite added.

"Well thank you for letting me know

sunshine.  I'm just happy for the chance to see you again.  You are still the sparkle in my eye. I trust that you will be successful on this mission and I know that you will be back home soon.  By the way, how are you enjoying the human experience?  I know that they are one of my more peculiar creations, but there is still much that you can learn from them.  Have they taught you anything?" Rah asked.

"They have indeed dad.  They are full of contradictions.  They don't seem too interested in evolving as much as many of the other beings.  They seem imprisoned by their emotions.  They also have a difficult time understanding love," Afro-dite eagerly shared hoping that Rah had some form of an explanation for humanity's peculiar behavior.

"Yes, all of what you have observed is correct.  The humans are flawed in that way. However, it is up to them to change those things.  I created them to evolve only by their own free will.  However, most of them have given that up," Rah explained.

"Well I understand dad and nonetheless, I will continue to carry out my mission and sooner rather than later I'll be back home once again!" Afro-dite said and with that she was gone.

Rah was so happy to see his daughter and how mature and responsible she was becoming. He saw that she was really proving herself capable and trustworthy of handling important, difficult missions. However, from what she told him he had some great concerns. He wasn't sure if she would be able to fully handle it on her own.

Nonetheless, he believed in her. In fact, he had to as there was no one else that he trusted enough to tell them what was going on. So he kept his secret and for once honored his daughter's wishes and put his trust in her.

Back on earth Afro-dite had a smile as

bright as sunshine that emitted pure joy. Upon seeing how proud her father was of her she had all the encouragement that she needed to successfully complete her mission.

The next couple of days were uneventful. However, the third day was anything but. Afro-dite had another run-in with the children who were teasing her about her hair. It seemed the girls had taken Afro-dite's kindness the other day for weakness as they began to act more boldly.

# Twenty-Three

That Monday, as was usually the case, Afro-dite had her hair in a huge afro. She was on her way to school when some of the girls that often teased her ran up behind her. There were four of them. They all walked to and from to school together everyday. They were all about the same age as Afro-dite. In fact, one of the more quiet ones was in her homeroom.

Her name was Tara. Tara was short, dark complexioned with short, dark brown hair which was usually braided with multi-colored beads at the ends. Tara didn't seem to belong with the group of girls. They were all bullies while Tara was more of a bookworm.

When she wasn't with the other girls Ayana, Liz and Kimberly she quite the model student. Afro-dite couldn't really figure her out, which seemed to be the running theme when it came to Afro-dite's understanding of humans. There was much about them that didn't quite make sense.

"Man you can see the world in her hair. Look at it!" pointed Ayana who was usually fairly quiet.

"I know right! The birds will probably think it's their bird nest. Let's put some bird seeds in there for when they get back," another girl name Kimberly taunted as she grabbed a paper bag from her back pack.

Then quietly inching closer up behind Afro-dite Kimberly threw a handful of sunflower of seeds into Afro-dite's hair! Because they were shelled the seeds had gotten all into Afro-dite's afro.

The other children roared with laughter. Some were being dramatic falling on the ground laughing.   Others were surrounding Afro-dite and pointing their fingers at her. While others yelled out rude remarks to Afro-dite.

Afro-dite, feeling her humanity rise, was enraged.  There was no reason for Kimberly to have done such a thing except from pure hatred and for that she would have to pay.

However, Afro-dite knew that by striking out at the children she ran the risk of possibly blowing her cover.  Her response would likely be something involving her powers, which would undoubtedly expose her true identity. She didn't want to do that so she tried with all of her might to calm the rage welling up inside of her.

She knew that if she gave into the rage her cover would be blown and she would not be able to successfully complete her mission. Aside from that it was too human a thing to do and that was just too beneath her as a primordial being.

Nonetheless, despite her efforts, around her the wind began to pick up speed. Leaves began to blow all around, the skies began to darken and the temperature got warmer. It was happening, Afro-dite was giving in to the rage despite all of her efforts not to!

She tried her best to focus on calming the storm that was brewing inside of her. Meanwhile, the girls were all standing around still laughing at her. Afro-dite just stood there, closed her eyes, silenced the noise around her and focused on staying peaceful.

As she focused and began to get a handle on her emotions the skies slowly began to brighten again, the winds lost speed and the temperature went back to normal. Meanwhile, the children were still laughing and pointing at her as if what they had just witnessed the funniest thing in existence.

Nonetheless, having once again returning to her calm Afro-dite parted her lips to speak. Curious about what she would say the children instantly became quiet. They had never heard Afro-dite speak and were more than anxious to finally hear her voice.

"Is your problem with me really about me or is there something that you really don't like about yourself?" Afro-dite asked.

"What?" Kimberly snapped.

"I'm sure you heard me. I can see that you're quite full of yourself, but that shouldn't stop your ears from working," Afro-dite answered sharply.

"Who are you talking to?" Kimberly fumed getting visibly more upset.

"Well as full as you are of yourself you tell me who else *would* I be talking to?" Afro-dite replied smugly.

"Girl you better go ahead unless you want more!" Kimberly winced.

"Oh is that so?  I didn't think you had anything to give anyone else.  Seems it's all about you Miss Full of Herself.  I mean isn't that what all this is about? Your teasing me I mean? Isn't your teasing about how much better you think you are than me?" Afro-dite continued before pausing.

"Or is it that you really don't like yourself and so you're taking it out on me?  Or is it that you just don't have anything better to do with your time?" Afro-dite asked before pausing again.

Kimberly stood frozen by her own embarrassment.

"Well I *do* have better things to do with *my* time and *you* are not one of them!" Afro-dite went on.  Then, with that she turned to walk away.

Overcome with fear, panic and shame Kimberly quickly ran up behind Afro-dite getting right up on her nearly inches away from her face.

"Girl I'll crush you! Say all that mess again! Say it right now!" Kimberly challenged.

"Oh really? Well if that was true you would have done that by now. And what exactly are you crushing me for? I didn't make you who you are and if crushing me is gonna make you feel better about the loser that you are then by all means take your best shot. But before you do you better ask yourself if it's worth it," Afro-dite snapped back holding her ground.

By then a large crowd of children had gathered around expecting a fight to break out at any moment.

"Don't take your frustration with yourself out on me. Find some better way to spend your time. I mean I'm glad that you find me just that interesting and all, but I know there must be way more interesting things in your life. I can't be that much of the superstar in your life or can I? Afro-dite said drawing Kimberly in for the kill.

"Well I didn't know that nappy headed people had so much to say. I guess under all those naps you really do have a brain hunh?" Kimberly taunted.

"Maybe... and it's also clear that nappy-headed people have *quite* the brain up under *all* the naps because if what you just said is the smartest thing that non-nappy-headed people have to say then I'll gladly keep my naps!" Afro-dite replied.

The children roared. They were all pointing at Kimberly laughing, some even bent over in laughter.

"Girl go somewhere and find a straightening comb!" Kimberly struck back.

"Why should I? It hasn't helped you any. You're all straightened and neat on the outside, but whatever is going on in the inside is just one big ole mess!" Afro-dite snapped back.

Again the children's laughter rang throughout the street.

"But I know what it is. Your life is just that boring and I'm the best part of it. I know. If that wasn't true you would have better things to do besides pick on me everyday. Are you that bored with your own life? Do you hate who you are that much? I get it though because if that was my miserable existence I might feel the same way. Anyway, I hope that what you just did makes the rest of your life wonderful. After all I'm sure doing hurtful things to people will bring you a really rewarding life and will probably make all of your dreams come true."

Afro-dite said.    Then with that she walked away.

Kimberly and the rest of the children all stood around speechless, not knowing what to say as they watched Afro-dite casually stroll away.

# Twenty-Four

Standing up to Kimberly was the best move that Afro-dite could have made because ever since that day she didn't have anymore issues with the kids teasing her. It seemed that using her mouth as a weapon was her saving grace. Contrary to her beliefs she realized that she didn't have to use her powers to solve all of her problems. Besides that, doing so would have certainly ruined her cover.

The rest of the day was uneventful and her day at school as well as the walk home went without a glitch. Though the same could not be said for what happened later that night as everyone else slept and Afro-dite explored the other realms.

As was the usual, that night Afro-dite

started to explore some of the other lower realms besides the physical realm. She started with the spiritual, auric and akashic realms trying to learn more about the identity of the who was behind using the humans to channel power.

One thing that bothered Afro-dite about the whole thing was how they were hiding behind the humans. It was a very wimpish thing to do and it definitely wasn't something that a primordial being would do.

It seemed rather childish so Afro-dite was beginning to consider that it might have been a god who was behind it. They were known among the more highly evolved to be quite childish as they weren't too much more evolved than the humans. However, she had her doubts about it being a god because they weren't powerful enough to go up against a primordial being and she couldn't imagine that they would ever be bold enough to try.

It was possible that it was a titan because they wanted to evolve to the next level, which was that of the primordial beings. Yet, Afro-dite thought to herself that it still didn't make sense because doing such a thing wasn't the way of a titan. Besides that, it was a childish manner of being that would never even allow one to gain access to the level of a primordial being.

This all led Afro-dite right back where she started, which was having not a clue as to who could be trying to take her father down. So she wandered through the lower realms using her power of magnetism to draw another clue to her.

Then, as was usually the case when she used her power of magnetism another clue came to her. She had just closed her eyes and shifted her consciousness to the Akashic realm when she saw what appeared to be a huge web.

The web seemed to go on forever. Afro-dite looked up and she saw that the web extended as far as she could see. She looked down, side to side from all angles and she saw the same thing.

It was like nothing she had ever before seen. Curious to see if was similar to a spider's web Afro-dite reached out to touch the web and to her surprise it was *very* similar to a spider's web. Then she tried to pull her hand back, but it was as if the web was sucking her in!

Afro-dite began to study the energy field of the web and noticed that it was identical to the one on the hair weave and the planet Earth. It had the exact same grid patterns and power centers. Afro-dite knew that she had come across another clue and that she was closer than ever to identifying who was after Rah.

Suddenly, as Afro-dite began to try to figure out what the web symbolized and what it meant the web began to attack her! It came.....

ALIVE!!!

Knowing that she was in the Akashic realm Afro-dite wondered whether she was in an illusion. It wasn't something typical of that realm, but as weird as things had gotten Afro-dite didn't discount anything. Besides that, the Akashic realm was nothing like the physical realm so anything was possible.

The Akashic realm was sort of like a library. It was a realm where all the memories from all the realms of consciousness were kept. Afro-dite wondered who the memory of the web belonged to.

Then as she pondered that the web began to attack her more violently. Though, unlike a spider's web, the web that was attacking Afro-dite was not coated with a sticky substance. Instead, it was coated with a mind altering substance that was injecting itself into Afro-dite's mind.

Before she knew it Afro-dite was in another realm. She had not willed herself to go to there, but the substance on the web somehow forced her into the shift.

# Twenty-Five

Looking around with a look of confusion Afro-dite quickly tried to assess where she had been brought to. Then when she looked up she saw the brightest shining sun that she'd ever seen.

Her father was the creator of all suns. However, as she read the energy field of the sun she saw that it was not of her father's creation. She wondered who else had been capable of doing such a thing. As far as she knew no one other than Rah had the power to create suns.

Afro-dite knew that she was onto a huge clue. Whoever had created the web was the same being that had created the sun as well as the weaves. In that moment she was more convinced than ever that it was a lower being.

She just didn't know if it was one of the titans or one of the gods.

What she *did* know was that it was not a primordial being because they were just as powerful as Rah. They just had powers unique to his. Nonetheless, they didn't have anything to prove.

Whoever was behind the whole scheme was definitely someone who had something to prove. The whole thing reeked of someone's ego. It reeked of someone needing to feel important. It reeked of someone needing to be noticed. Someone who needed to feel as bright as the sun about themself was behind the whole thing. Someone who needed to feel mighty was behind it.

Just then, having identified one more piece to the puzzle and desiring to return to the physical realm Afro-dite went to shift her consciousness back to the human realm and nothing happened. She closed her eyes and tried again, but still nothing.  She tried several more times all to no avail.

It seemed that something or someone was preventing Afro-dite from returning.  She knew that it had to be the mysterious being behind the plot to kill her father.  They may have even have known about her being there.  They definitely had taken the time to guard the realm against her powers so it wasn't too far fetched.

As a primordial being her powers were very unique.  Though there were several powers that all primordial beings shared the way the powers worked was unique to the individual being.  So whoever created the realm made it knowing that *she* would come there.

Feeling a sense of urgency to return more than ever and refusing to give up Afro-dite decided to give it another try.  She closed her eyes and really concentrated on shifting back using her primordial power of teleportation. However, rather than doing what she had done all the other times before in using only her own powers she channeled her parents powers as well.

Even that did not work at first so she had to try several more times. Finally, the fourth time she added her power of destruction to destroy the realm that she was stuck in. Her power of destruction was one that she very rarely invoked because it was often too difficult for her to come back from it.

Whenever she used her power of destruction it caused her to shift into her other self and it was a version of Afro-dite that was often unstoppable. Knowing that Afro-dite used only a small amount of her destructive power to take down the realm.

Finally, back into her human body Afro-dite opened her eyes and sat upright. The Akashic realm had definitely given her another crucial piece of the puzzle. It also let her know that the traitor must have been expecting someone to track them there and the someone that they expected was Afro-dite, but how? How could they have known that *she* would come.

It seemed that whoever it was always was a few steps ahead of Afro-dite so she had to figure out a way to get a few steps ahead of them for a change. However, they'd been so good at hiding that she wondered if she'd ever be able to. They were more hidden then even Rah at the moment. Everyone left a trail of some sort, but this person was almost invisible. It was like they were a ghost of sorts.

Afro-dite sat in the bed for the remainder of the night deep in thought. She went through everything that had happened thus far over and over and over again in her head. Then she called forth her powers of magnetism again to help her to figure things out.

Then the next morning it suddenly came

to her.  She figured out who the traitor was, or rather who they were disguised as!

# Twenty-Six

Afro-dite couldn't believe that she hadn't realized it sooner. The traitor had been there all along. They had been there quietly taunting her, teasing her and laughing at how clueless she was as to their true identity. They were the thing in the human realm that didn't quite belong, the subtle detail that could easily be overlooked, the unnoticeable flaw.

All of this time they were there. They even had others in place to distract Afro-dite from noticing them. They had others in place to overwhelm Afro-dite with her humanness so that she got thrown off of their scent.

They had somehow identified Afro-dite from the start, from the day of her arrival. They knew of her coming and had put themself in place just in time to watch her every move.

It was Tara, the quiet one, the little girl that didn't quite fit in with the others! Tara was the silent leader. She was the one whose commands the others followed.

Afro-dite couldn't believe that she hadn't noticed earlier. It was always the quiet ones, the ones who sat back and just observed that had to be watched. That was who Tara was. The others would tease, but Tara would never say a word.

Then, when Afro-dite thought about it she remembered that she'd also seen Tara that day at the beauty supply store. Tara seemed to know the lady at the register, the one who definitely had something to do with the weaves.

Thoughts were running through Afro-dite's mind a million miles per minute. She wanted to know what the little girl's connection was to the higher realm? She too was disguising herself as a human, but Afro-dite wanted to know who she truly was.

Afro-dite also wanted to know how Tara and the lady in the beauty supply store were connected and what their plans were for the weaves?  She wanted to know how they were able to track her to the Akashic realm?  How they were always 5 steps ahead of her?

It was time for Afro-dite to get 10 steps ahead of them!  That meant that she had to figure out the little girl's true identity and she had to do so without her knowing.

Afro-dite also had to figure out how the little girl had gotten onto the planet past the quarantine that Rah had set up.  It had many times proven itself full proof and Afro-dite couldn't imagine how they got around it.

Later that day while Jackie was cooking

dinner Afro-dite was sitting in the living room pretending to watch television though deep in thought about what was going on when suddenly something happened that blew her mind! She looked up and couldn't believe who was standing in her aunt's house!

# Twenty-Seven

Standing right before her with the most cunning smile was Tara! Posing as a 'friend' of Afro-dite's Tara had knocked on the door and asked Jackie if Afro-dite could come out and play.

How did Tara know where Afro-dite lived? It was as if Tara was tapped into Afro-dite's thoughts. Her timing was too good to be coincidental. More than that since Tara knew that Afro-dite wouldn't dare risk blowing her cover by attacking her she knew that she was safe making such a bold move. She also knew the best way to make the first move was by confronting Afro-dite and drawing her in, which was exactly what she did.

Interrupting Jackie as she was telling

Tara that she would go and see if Afro-dite wanted to come out, Afro-dite calmly walked over to the door and told Jackie that she did in fact want to go outside. She then walked past Jackie out the door giving Jackie a reassuring look to let her know that all was well so that Jackie would close the door and go back into the house.

Things were bound to get ugly and Afro-dite didn't dare want any humans, let alone Jackie to witness it. It was kind of an unspoken rule that the more highly evolved never exposed their powers to the natives of the realms they visited. It tended to throw the balance of things way off in such a way that it impacted all of the realms. What happened in one realm impacted all of the realms. It seemed that even Tara respected that rule despite her having defied many of the others.

Yet, the second Jackie closed the door Afro-dite began to feel rage beginning to rise up within her as she inched closer to Tara. She wanted to more closely examine her energetic field to see if there was anything familiar about it.

"Show yourself!" Afro-dite commanded.

"I am. I have nothing to hide. In fact, I have been in plain sight since you got here," Tara replied.

"What are you called? What is your true form?" Afro-dite asked as she tried to see what Tara's true form was for herself. Yet something was blocking her from seeing it.

As a primordial being there were no cloaking powers that she could not see through. So she could not understand what it was that was preventing her from seeing Tara's true identity.

Just then Afro-dite realized what it was. It was magical!

"You are.... the magician! This is your magic. Where did you learn such magic?" Afro-dite asked.

"Oh little girl these are powers. Magic is child's play. You high and mighty primordial beings in all of your arrogance *would* think that powers were only reserved for *you*. Well let me tell you... they aren't. Not only do I have powers, but the powers I have are far greater than anything in the universe. Right this very instant your father is learning that very hard lesson. As a matter of fact, how is oh Daddy oh?" Tara sneered with a sly grin.

Growing agitated by Tara's overconfidence in her abilities Afro-dite replied, "Oh, is that so? Well I doubt your so-called 'powers' are all that great since I've already broken through them. You're no threat to my father or me. And if anyone is being arrogant it's you in deluding yourself into thinking that you are more powerful than a primordial. You must have some sort of a death wish to even think that you can go up against us and the nerve of you to come here and threaten his beloved humans!"

"Oh I am not at all mistaken about the strength of my powers and you will soon see that! Oh and by the way, the name's Weava! Tara is the scared little girl who hides behind bullies. I don't hide behind anyone. I guess you can't say the same daddy's girl!" Tara taunted as she smiled then pointed her finger to Afro-dite's apartment door.

Just then the door opened and out walked Jackie and Candi seemingly under Weava's control. When Afro-dite looked at them she saw that the energy field around their head was bright red and their eyes were blood red! In fact, their eyes looked just like the warrior's eyes who had attacked the guests at Afro-dite's birthday party when the magician sent them all to Mars.

Weava had done something similar and

by then Afro-dite realized that Weava was in fact, the magician. She had even come to her birthday party in a disguise because she appeared then as a man. Afro-dite then realized that Weave had been planning the whole thing since the party. In fact, she used the party as a test run.

As Afro-dite began to put all the pieces together Jackie and Candi were heading her way and positioning themselves to attack. She didn't want to hurt them as she knew that they were being controlled by Weava.

"So as you can see my powers are everywhere. You can't escape them and you can't defeat them! How about we let you see that for yourself?" Weava said motioning with her hand for Jackie and Candi to attack.

Wanting to ensure that she did everything that she could to avoid hurting them Afro-dite decided to flee until she had time to come up with a plan to stop Weava from controlling them.    So using her power of teleportation Afro-dite teleported herself to the rooftop of the building where she could take a moment to think and come up with a plan.

# Twenty-Eight

On the rooftop Afro-dite quickly tried to come up with a plan. She knew that she was at a great disadvantage as Weava had thousands of innocents at her disposal.

She used humans as mere pawns in her sick chess game and had absolutely no regard for their lives. Afro-dite knew that her father would have been devastated if his humans were destroyed knowing that they were innocent. So in order to get to Weava Afro-dite would have to come up with a way to do so without harming any innocent humans.

She knew that she didn't have much time because Weava had made an army of humans and she had to act quickly before that army grew any larger. Then, Afro-dite came up with a plan.

She remembered that Weava was controlling the women by way of the weaves in their hair.  So Afro-dite just needed to come up with a way to get the weaves out of their hair.  However, she had no idea how she would do that.  The women were obsessed with wearing weaves.  Even little girls had Weava's hair weaved into their own as braids.

As long as Weava's hair controlled the masses any and everyone was a potential enemy.  Weava had woven quite the web of deceit.  She had convinced women that their own natural beauty was not good enough.  She had deceived them into believing that their beauty came from something outside of themselves.  Weava convinced them that beauty was something that had to be purchased in a beauty supply store.

Afro-dite had to convince them otherwise.  She had to prove to them that they were beautiful just the way they were naturally.

Then she figured it out!   She would defeat Weava by simply reminding women that beauty did not have to be bought and that it was something that each of them possessed. She figured out the perfect way to do just that.

Later that night, Afro-dite returned home. Uncertain as to whether Jackie and Candi were still under Weava's spell or not she first shape-shifted as a small table plant then used her power of magnetism to get Alan to bring her home to Jackie who set her on the dining room table.

Once inside Afro-dite saw that they were no longer under Weava's spell.   In fact, they were all in the living room trying to figure out where *she* was.   It seemed they had no memory of being under Weava's control.   So Afro-dite teleported herself outside of the door then shape-shifted back into her human body.

After taking a few seconds to come up

with her cover story Afro-dite knocked on the door.   Jackie anxiously answered the door, hugging Afro-dite tightly and greeting her warmly as she enters the apartment.

"Where have you been little girl?  We've been looking everywhere for you.  No one knew anything about that little girl you went to play with earlier so we didn't know where you were," Jackie said with a look of concern.

"Oh we went to her house to play.  She lives two buildings down," Afro-dite answered.

"Ok well next time just let us know where you're going because we were worried sick," Jackie said closing the door behind Afro-dite.

When Afro-dite got inside she saw that the family was preparing to eat and had apparently been waiting for her.  Carla ran up and hugged Afro-dite also apparently relieved that she was back.

Once Afro-dite got settled in and everyone had gotten cleaned up they all had dinner. Afro-dite spent the rest of the evening ironing out the details of her plans. She was anxious for bedtime so that she could get to work. Then as soon as everyone was asleep she did just that.

# Twenty-Nine

Afro-dite didn't waste anytime. She wasn't sure how she was doing it, but Weava was always a few steps ahead of her and she wanted to make sure that didn't happen again.

While everyone slept Afro-dite went into the under realm. The under realm was a lot like the Akashic realm. It was where all human thoughts, beliefs and emotions were recorded. It was like an underground library.

Afro-dite teleported there and quickly went to work on locating the human beliefs about beauty. She used her power of magnetism to speed things up a bit and in no time she had located all of the records.

Next, she re-wrote the beliefs and just as she was about to seal the records Weava showed up.  Afro-dite had not planned for Weava to find her there.  However, she was prepared to defend against Weava nonetheless.

There were no humans around to maintain a cover for so she was free to wield her powers as she pleased.  In the under realm Afro-dite was free to exist in her natural form.

So immediately upon seeing Weava Afro-dite struck her with a ball of hot gas.  As the daughter of Rah who possessed all of the power of the sun Afro-dite was able to access that same energy and she did so with great skill.

However, Weava seemed unaffected. Afro-dite looked at her energy field and saw that the Weava before her wasn't actually Weava.  Instead, she was a hologram.  It was another one of Weava's illusions.

Unable to attack a hologram Afro-dite

tried attacking Weava another way. She invoked her power of magnetism and drew to her all of the recorded beliefs about weaves. When the records came forth she quickly struck them with an energy ball.

Suddenly Weava appeared in full form yelling, "What have you done? That was my life's work! Do you know how hard I worked to get those humans to trust me enough to harness those beliefs. You'll pay for that little girl and you'll pay dearly!"

With that Weava was gone. Afro-dite stood beaming with a smile as wide as the universe pleased with her success. She'd done it. She'd broken the link of control that Weava had over the humans and she was overjoyed.

Nonetheless, she knew that the battle had not yet been won and that Weava would still have to be destroyed. So she completed the task at hand then sealed up the recorded beliefs about beauty. Once she finished she left the under realm and returned back to her human body.

As she laid in the bed she started to work on the next part of her plan. She knew that Weava would be back and that she had to be ready for her. That meant that she had to be prepared to take Weava out when the time came because there would probably not be another opportunity.

# Thirty

The next morning Afro-dite was anxious to see how humans would respond to the changes made to their beliefs about beauty and weaves. She was also curious to see if Weava would show up as Tara for school.

As expected, that morning beauty was in the air. Jackie and Candi were practically singing their own praises all morning. Afro-dite overheard them discussing wanting to 'go natural' and how they needed to start getting to know their own hair.

Afro-dite couldn't have been happier. She wanted to allow people to come into knowledge of their inner beauty on their own free will, but time did not allow as Weava was fast on her heels. So she had to act fast.

Soon it was time to head to school so Afro-dite grabbed her backpack and headed out the door. She was more than ready for Weava. She had already set a plan to get rid of her once and for all.

When she got downstairs she saw the usual crew walking together with the exception of Weava. She looked around and didn't see Weava anywhere. She wondered what Weava was up to. She kept walking to school nonetheless. She knew that Weava was too full of herself to be run off that easily. So she waited.

The school day came and went and there was no sign of Weava. In fact, several days had passed and there wasn't a single hint of Weava's presence anywhere.

Meanwhile, the humans were really coming into loving their own natural beauty. There were reports that the new natural hair craze was spreading like wild fire. Afro-dite couldn't have been more pleased with her work.  She figured that once she got rid of Weava she would have killed two birds with one stone.  Her father would be so proud.

Then, like clockwork Weava struck again interrupting Afro-dite's thoughts.

# Thirty-One

Appearing in the Astral realm where Afro-dite was hanging out deep in thought Weava appeared as cocky as ever.

"Well what do we have here? A happy-go-lucky primordial who thinks she's won," Weava sneered.

"Not surprised to see you here. So what took you so long?" Afro-dite inquired.

"Well I thought *you* would know that. Shouldn't an all-knowing primordial being like yourself know these things? Hmph, I guess when you hang out in the clouds so much you're bound to lose touch with what's going on in the real world. Then again what is real, especially in this holographic reality that we call the human life?" Weava said smiling.

Realizing what Weava was hinting around at Afro-dite quickly returned to the human realm. She came back to her human body to find that humanity was in a state of pure chaos.

Weava had done the unthinkable. She had gone too far. The stakes were then higher than ever and Afro-dite was out for blood. She was determined more than ever to make Weava pay.

Afro-dite had returned to find that Weava had bound the entire planet into one, huge web-like weave. The skies were dark and all that you could see were long strands of hair weaves.

Yet, Weava didn't stop there. There were strands of weave, which extended from the web and connected to every human brain, man, woman and child. There were some humans who were bound together in bunches serving as power centers on what seemed to be one huge energy grid.

Then to Afro-dite's surprise the power being channeled from the energy grid was aimed straight at Sirius! Weava was using the power obtained from the human brains to launch an attack on her home planet Sirius!

# Thirty-Two

Afro-dite had to act quickly to help save her planet. Even with all of the primordials there she didn't know if even they were powerful enough to ward off such an attack. She also knew that her father was depending on her to end the attack from Earth so she had to do something quick or else all would be lost!

Yet, before Afro-dite could respond to the problems-at-hand Weava was attacking her with smaller distractions. Again controlling humanity, Weava had programmed the humans to attack Afro-dite. She had to decide between returning home to fight Weava alongside her family or battling Weava on her own down on Earth.

If she didn't defeat Weava on Earth there was a chance that Weava would get away. On the other hand, if she didn't return home to help her family there was a chance that the home of the primordials would be destroyed.

Sirius was the most ancient star system in existence and there was no way that Afro-dite was going to let Weava destroy it. Besides that, there was no way that Afro-dite was going to lose her family at the hands of Weava.

Feeling the rage welling up inside of her Afro-dite began to turn into the Destructress whom all called Sekhem. Sekhem, was the her other half and was a fierce warrior primordial being whose rage could destroy entire planets and all life in its path.

It was a side of Afro-dite that never needed to come out unless absolutely necessary and as a last resort. Once Sekhem was unleashed the only one that could calm her was Rah and since Rah was occupied defending Sirius there was no telling what would become of Sekhem's destructive force. It wasn't the time to unleash Sekhem who was an unstoppable force so Afro-dite tried with all of her might to calm herself down.

She knew that if she turned into Sekhem all of humanity would be destroyed. So Afro-dite closed her eyes and channeled the strength of her mother and father to keep Sekhem bound.

# Thirty-Three

As Afro-dite tried with everything in her might to keep Sekhem bound it was to no avail. Sekhem was getting stronger by the minute though Afro-dite tried with everything in her to push through.

In doing so she heard the voice of her father speak to her saying, "Afro-dite, Afro-dite…. You don't need her right now. You can defeat Weava on your own. You have the power to defeat her. Believe in yourself. I believe in you and I trust that you can. *You* must know that you can."

Hearing the voice of Rah instantly soothed Afro-dite's mind and calmed her rage. Rah believed in her ability and so did she. She came back into herself looked around at the chaos that was going on around her and had the most intense feeling of calm. It was a space of peace in the eye of Weava's storm.

Having gained more insight from her own invocation of peace Afro-dite was able to see things more clearly. She was able to see with the eye of Rah! The eye of Rah was a power that only she possessed as he knew that she was the only one powerful enough to contain its light. Afro-dite was back in control and everything was crystal clear.

Through the eyes of Rah she saw that Weava's energy grid was very similar what she, herself had done at Majestic Forest. So Afro-dite quickly teleported herself there to recharge. She had a plan. She needed to infuse all the power that she could into her hair.

Humanity was on the verge of being destroyed. Yet, in order to save them Afro-dite had to stay focused. So the instant that she arrived at Majestic Forest the forest bonded with her hair and she felt the familiar surge of energy begin to flood her body. The moment it was done Afro-dite returned to Earth.

She had to get rid of Weava once and for all so rather than try to separate the humans from the weaves Afro-dite had another plan in mind. Since the humans were so connected to the weave to the point of having an unbreakable loyalty to it such that they were prepared to defend it with their lives Afro-dite had to do something unexpected.

Their eyes were blood red and they were blood-thirsty, but only for Afro-dite's blood. She looked into their eyes and saw only hate. All love was gone. The had no love for themselves. They had no love for life. In that moment all they knew was the hate-filled thoughts that Weava and filled their heads with by way of her venomous weaves.

The moment they saw Afro-dite they all came charging for her. Unlike the previous time in the apartment building, Afro-dite did not flee.  She stood her ground.

Then as the humans came charging towards her looking like strands of hair with poisonous arrow tips Afro-dite had caused her hair to produce an oil.  The oil was was both a medicine and a poison.

Since the weaves were all connected to Weava Afro-dite had made it so the oil healed the humans severing the hold that the Weava's weave had on their minds.  At the same time, the oil was poisonous to Weava.

As Afro-dite invoked the oil to surface her afro became larger than life.  It looked just like it did in the Majestic Forest.  Her afro was so big that is covered the earth like a cap.

For every strand of weave there were 10 strands of Afro-dite's hair.  Afro-dite's hair then began to reproduce new strands that sprung up like weeds all across the Earth.  Unable to grow and reproduce, the strands of weave were outnumbered.

Once the planet was covered with Afro-dite's hair up sprang the healing oils. The oils covered the planet like a flood and instantly healed every human in it's path. By the thousands Afro-dite began to see the humans turn back to normal and as they did strands of weave connected to them fizzled into nothing and disappeared.

Meanwhile, Afro-dite still had to locate Weava. She quickly used her power of magnetism to bring Weava to her before she had a chance to escape. Instantly Weava appeared.

# Thirty-Four

"You think you've won! You may have won the battle, but I assure you we'll win the war. You haven't seen the last of me Afro-dite!" Weava said smugly.

"Oh yeah," Afro-dite replied, "I doubt that. There won't be a comeback for what I have planned for you. There's this new hot oil treatment that I recently created that is changing the entire hair business as we know it. You should give it a try."

"Yeah give it your best shot little girl!" Weava sneered.

Then, Afro-dite commanded a bunch of her hair strands to pour the oil on Weava, but Weava was bobbing and weaving too quickly. Afro-dite's strands could not catch her.

"Ha ha ha! You can't catch me I'm the Weave Girl Bandit!" Weava teased as she continued to evade the hair strands.

Just then Afro-dite commanded several bunches of hair strands to surround Weava stopping Weava dead in her tracks. Weava had no where to run. She couldn't go up or down as there were strands of Afro-dite's hair above her head, beneath her feet and surrounding her.

"Well I guess you got me. But you still haven't won. Oh the tangled webs we weave when we try to deceive. See you in another lifetime primordial one," Weava said as she began to fizzle away.

Along with her fizzled away the remaining strands of weave. Then all across the planet humans began to return to normal. The healing oil removed all traces of humanity's memory of Weava's control over them and all that had transpired.

Afro-dite didn't want to disrupt the balance of things across the other realms by having humans remember all that had just happened. She also didn't need her true identity to be know or her powers exposed. So she took the necessary steps to cover her tracks. She gathered herself and returned to Jackie's house to maintain her cover.

As she looked at the glow illuminating from each human face Afro-dite smiled to herself happy to have successfully completed the mission and happy to have given humanity the gift of self-love.

Seeing them love their natural selves was the greatest reward that she could have ever asked for. She couldn't wait to see the look on her father's face when she reported back to him. In face, getting back to Sirius was all that she could think about. She was worried and needed to see if her family was okay.

# Thirty-Five

Afro-dite couldn't wait to report back to Rah. Nighttime couldn't arrive fast enough. She was more anxious than ever to go to bed that night and for everyone else to go to sleep.

Seemingly exhausted from the night's events everyone went to bed early and in no time they were all fast asleep. Afro-dite took full advantage of it and made her way home to Sirius.

However, when she arrived what she saw did not at all bring her joy. Sirius had been dealt some devastating blows from Weava's attack. There were injured primordial beings lying about everywhere. Pockets of the planet were exploding and other parts were quaking.

Frantic, Afro-dite went to find her

parents.  When she arrived what she saw dealt her an even more devastating blow.  Her father was standing over her mother looking distraught as ever.  Afro-dite ran over to him and hugged him tightly.

"Dad what happened to mom?" Afro-dite shrieked.

"Oh dear daughter you made it back! Did you defeat her?  Your mother will be fine. We will all be fine," Rah said assuringly.

"I did defeat her dad.  I heard your voice and I did it.  I didn't know that she caused so much destruction here though.  What happened to mom?" Afro-dite asked again with a worried look on her face.

"Your mother was hit by an energy bolt. I tried to intercept it but there were too many coming at once and I couldn't stop them all. Nonetheless, I was able to break it's impact so that it merely grazed her.  She will be fine.  She just needs some time to heal. At any rate I am very pleased with you my sunshine. You did exactly what I knew you could do," Rah said endearingly.

"I couldn't have done it without you dad, you and mom. I almost came back here to help here and it was a difficult choice not to abandon the mission," Afro-dite said. "But I remembered what you said," she added.

"Oh no dear. You never abandon a mission. If I give you a mission it's because I need you fighting from that side. You made the right choice just as I knew you would sunshine. I saw everything from here and you faced some tough choices. I know that you wanted to abandon humanity, but it's not yet time for their end. I knew that in the end you would see that," Rah said.

"I love you dad. Thank you for believing in me. There were times when I doubted that and I'm sorry," Afro-dite said hugging Rah once again.

It was time for the big clean up so Afro-dite helped get her mother comfortable and then called for the healers to come and tend to her. Rah called for the cleaners and in no time Sirius was back stronger than ever.

# Thirty-Six

Meanwhile, on Earth life went on as usual. Afro-dite made sure that the humans had no memory of what happened. They were still hair obsessed and many of them still wore hair weaves. However, a huge majority of them had embraced their natural beauty and started to wear their own natural hair. In fact, there was a new craze and it was that being all natural was beautiful.

Little girls no longer teased one another about their natural hair and everyone started to embrace the unique beauty that everyone had. Mother's no longer ventured doing their daughters' hair with dread. Natural beauty was seen as a prized possession.

As was Afro-dite's desire humanity had finally come to discover natural beauty on their own free will. They were their own inspiration and they discovered the beauty within. Afro-dite began to think that despite their many flaws there was hope for humanity after all. They were finally discovering the gift of self love.

It was the one gift that Rah gave them and it was his desire to see them realize it by way of their own free will. He was pleased to see that they were beginning to evolve. Afro-dite was pleased to be a part of making her dad's dream come true.

More than that she was happy about having successfully accomplished her first mission. She knew that she could do it all along and seeing it become a reality was her first step toward becoming the first of the next generation of great primordial creators.

Meanwhile, during her spare time she still enjoyed entertaining herself as a human being as part of Jackie's family. Going back and forth between realms gave Afro-dite an opportunity to grow as a primordial being in that it kept her humble. It also forced her to work harder at developing her powers while encased in a human body. It was that, which ended up making Afro-dite one of the most powerful primordial beings of all time.

She aspired to live up to her father's name and she worked nonstop on her journey to reaching his level of ascension.

Meanwhile, a new force was on the rise. As Afro-dite's powers grew so did it. It was a force that was enemy of the ancient primordial ones not friend and it was coming for them all with a vengeance!!

TO BE CONTINUED.....

If you enjoyed this book or received value from it in any way, then I'd like to ask you for a favor. Would you be kind enough to leave a review for this book on Amazon? It'd be greatly appreciated!

# About the Author....

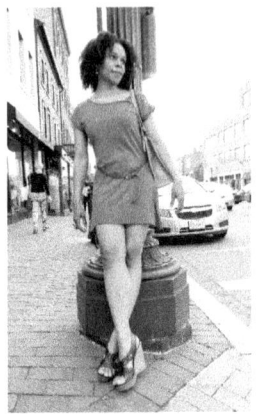

**Amirah Bellamy** is the board chair of Life Arts Institute. She is an artist of many crafts. She's been a writer for over 19 years, a yogi for over 9 years, a singer for over 15 years, nutritionista for over 16 years and has thoroughly enjoyed being mom to 2 beautiful children.

**To learn more about Amirah Bellamy**

**email… amirahbellamy@gmail.com**
                        **or**
**visit….. www.EthericRealmsInv.com**

# Other books written by this author....

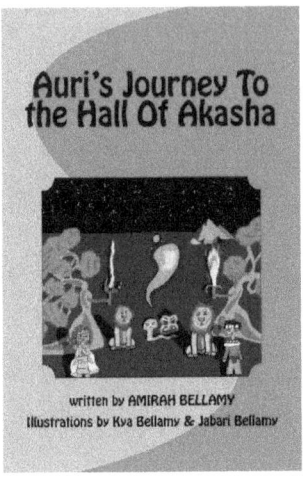